There's Always Hope

A Mother's Her-story of Multiple Chemical and
Electromagnetic Sensitivities

Adversity, Hope and Enlightenment

Linda Springer

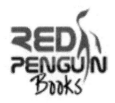

To my son Bret, my guru.

To my parents, Mel and Sylvia Springer, who never wavered in their support, commitment and love!

To my husband Ernie who was always there for me!

To all of the people suffering with EMS and MCS. May you find the answers to overcome your illness!

Contents

Part One

The Medical Journey

Breaking the Circuit

"Are we ready?" Ernie would yell to both Bret and me. I was in the living room laying on the pull out bed. Bret was sealed in his room, as he always was.

Step by step, we could hear Ernie lumber down the basement stairs, slow and deliberate, flashlight in hand.

Click by click, we would hear him switch off each circuit breaker until the entire house was enveloped in complete darkness and silence. No humming, buzzing, or electronic alert tones—just us—our breathing and hearts aching and beating for one another. Then Ernie would methodically ascend the stairs as Bret achieved a little bit of peace and drift off to sleep.

. . .

This was our evening ritual, once we knew of the extent of Bret's Electromagnetic Sensitivity (EMS). His was a medical condition that was previously unknown to us, but would impact all of our lives and turn our world upside down.

At Bret's request, we had to find a way to reduce his exposure to this agonizing energy flowing through his environment, and this nightly ritual was one small way to give him some temporary relief.

Life Before MCS/EMS

*I*t all seems as if it were a dream. But it wasn't—it resembled more of a nightmare! In 2010 we experienced a life-altering experience, one that affected the entire family. This book is my account of the story.

We are a family of three: my son Bret, my husband Ernie, and me, Linda.

We live in suburbia about 50 miles east of New York City, an average middle-class family living the Long Island life. Our life includes access to all the modern conveniences just minutes away, including car transportation with limited access to mass transit, multiple strip malls and shopping centers, good school districts, a generous and varied assortment of restaurants, and access to numerous beautiful sandy beaches, while only an hour away from Manhattan.

. . .

Long Island is a land mass on the Eastern Seaboard which juts out into the Atlantic Ocean and Long Island Sound off the coast of New York City. It holds the counties of Kings, Queens, Nassau, and Suffolk. Kings County (a.k.a. Brooklyn) and Queens County are part of New York City proper, while Nassau and Suffolk lie just outside the city boundaries. We live in a three-bedroom ranch house in Suffolk, the county farthest from the city. Our home is on the Ronkonkoma moraine, a glacier deposit which has created a rather hilly pastoral landscape. Benefitting from a temperate climate, we experience all four seasons, each with its unique characteristics. My parents lived nearby in Nassau County, while the rest of our immediate family was either out of state or pre-deceased us.

Both my husband and I work, and I am self-employed.

Who am I?

I have always had a deep love for the beach and the sea. When I was eight years old, I found a sea shell at Sunken Meadow State Park on the north shore of Long Island, and asked my Dad, "What is the name of this shell?" This led to a lifelong hobby of shell collecting for both myself and my Dad, which has generated one of the largest personal shell collections in the country.

. . .

We helped found the Long Island Shell Club in the mid-1970's, comprising of like-minded local shell collectors.

When collecting at the beach, one of the first things you need to know is, "When is low tide?" This provides the best opportunity to find seashells, and other marine life, that might have been submerged during high tide. The most opportune tide, the lowest of the low tides, is usually a full moon tide.

I am a naturalist, a bird watcher, grounded to the earth. My talents were put to use curating the Crane Collection, an extensive fossil and extant shell collection, at the Museum of Long Island Natural Sciences, located at the Earth and Space Science Building on the campus of SUNY Stony Brook (the State University of New York at Stony Brook). I also did grant work at the Museum, including a Pine Barrens exhibit, and my crowning achievement was co-authoring three field guides on Long Island's Woodlands, Wetlands, and Seashore. All of this was a dream come true! As I would be leading a field trip for the Museum, I'd say to myself, "Pinch me. I can't believe I am doing this, making my dreams come true."

I became pregnant with Bret in July 1986, during a trip to California and a tryout for the TV quiz show *Jeopardy*. I didn't pass the audition, so I teased that Bret was my "parting gift" for the *Jeopardy* tryout.

3

Bret

_____

*B*ret was an honor student, a Boy Scout and a musician.

When Bret was four, we enrolled him in T-ball. He played for two years, wasn't very good, and finally declared, "I love watching baseball, but I do not love playing it." That was the end of his T-ball and sports career.

Cub Scouts and Boy Scouts was a much better fit for him. He achieved the rank of "Star" through his participation, leadership, service and compilation of merit badges.

I also was able to contribute to the pack and troop and was a Scout Leader. My background as a naturalist was a huge plus when the Scouts strove to earn the many merit badges that are nature-related.

I remember when the Boy Scouts were having a large Jamboree at Great Adventure in Jackson Township, New Jersey. Bret asked, "Mom would you go so I can go on the big roller coasters with you?" I did, and it turned out that I was the only woman attending from the troop. When we arrived on Friday night, the leaders of our troop made sure my tent was strategically surrounded so there would be no trouble. The campground also had a line of porta potties, one with a paper plate taped to it that said "Women." By the next morning someone had ripped off the paper plate and the few women at the event no longer had a "private" bathroom.

On Saturday, we hiked into the Great Adventure theme park, and used their bathrooms to wash up. I asked Bret, "What's the first roller coaster you want to go on?" He replied, "I don't want to go on the big roller coasters." And so it goes.

Bret was strong-willed, and, on that particular day, had a fear of riding the roller coaster. It's a young person's prerogative to change his mind, I guess. If it isn't enjoyable, why should we do it? But we still had a lot of fun enjoying all of the other amenities Great Adventure offered.

· · ·

Bret was also a young man with musical talents and interests. A trumpet player going into high school, he came home at the end of ninth grade and said, "Mom, I want to learn how to play the French Horn! The band teacher asked for volunteers to move from trumpet to French Horn, and I volunteered." He was given the name of a private French Horn tutor and Bret immediately began to take private lessons. By working so hard and practicing endlessly, Bret received a glowing recommendation from his music teacher to audition for the Long Island Youth Orchestra. He earned a place on the Orchestra and played French Horn, second chair. The C.W. Post Campus of Long Island University hosted its practices and recitals. During this tenure, Bret was fortunate to travel with the Orchestra for five weeks to Australia, New Zealand, Tonga, and Samoa. Travel had clearly become an emerging passion. This exposure elicited an invitation for him to perform with the LIU college orchestra as well. Quite an honor for a high school student!

He regaled us with great stories about his five week trip. The Orchestra would perform and then meet with local children to educate them on music and their instruments. When the Youth Orchestra was in Samoa, they were treated like royalty. The Prime Minister hosted a dinner feast at the Robert Louis Stevenson House in their honor. It doesn't get much better than that!

With Bret's strong musical talent and his intellectual gifts (did I mention he is smart, too?), he received a full academic scholarship from George Mason University in Fairfax, Virginia. Loving his experiences in his high school band and orchestras, he chose to study Music Education. We visited as often as we could, and Bret came home on breaks.

For the first two years at GMU, Bret lived on campus, like an ordinary academic. For his junior year, determined to room with friends and expand his horizons, he chose to move off campus. The apartments were affectionately called "Camp Pyro," and they were a pig sty. His mattress was rescued from a garbage pick up in front of a nearby home. Yuck! At this time he also tried the vegan lifestyle, but it didn't quite work for him, causing an alarming and unhealthy weight fluctuation.

In college, Bret excelled academically, but he also decided that teaching music was not the career path he wished to pursue. The classroom students he met in his field studies lacked the zest for musical knowledge and the desire to learn that he found during his travels. He graduated with a bachelor's degree in music, but without a clear course for his future. Nevertheless, he remained optimistic for what was to come.

Little did he know that he soon would be horribly ill.

4

Melting Into The Couch

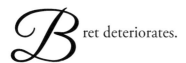ret deteriorates.

Bret came home from college in January 2010, looking pale and tired. He lay down on the couch and quickly deteriorated, almost as if he was being absorbed into the couch itself.

Visiting multiple doctors and recommended medical specialists provided no answers and a great deal of exasperation. We frequently heard the words, "Good luck. This is beyond our realm of expertise." If the medical field was unable to help us—then to whom do we turn?

And then, it got even worse.

· · ·

One doctor recommended that we should find an environmental specialist to work with. To him, the symptoms Bret was experiencing were all responses of his body to outside sources and stimuli. A doctor who specializes in environmental illnesses might be able to help. He recommended one, but it turned out she only worked with patients who got ill in the workplace.

Aha! It's an environmental issue! We had a path to follow! Now we had to do the homework.

When your son is sick and dying, the grief, worry and emotional devastation are unbearable. And a sense of overall hopelessness makes it definitely worse.

Bret displayed symptoms that were shocking to see, and certainly beyond any illness I had witnessed or heard of. Here are some of the symptoms and the "bandaids" I used to help his reactions:

1. A negative reaction to all chemicals. He went to visit a friend who happened to be using bleach. An encounter with bleach nearly killed Bret, and he passed out. He reacted violently to any perfumes, cleaners, laundry detergents, shampoos, soaps and toothpastes. I had to isolate

him to remove him from even a chance exposure to a wide variety of typical household products—and all of the above-mentioned. I found safer alternatives like Dr Bronner's soap and organic shampoos.

2. Electromagnetic sensitivity to most electrical impulses, including WiFi, high tension towers, refrigerators, TVs, radios, computers. He would have an agonizing pain in his head and abdominal area when he was exposed. I found that if he would ground his body to the earth, such as touching a tree, that that would literally ground him and release the pain. Eventually we chose to turn off all electricity in the house at night to give his body a rest. We'd unplug the refrigerator and use a cooler for the bare essentials—and ate out a lot.

3. An inability to read because the acid in the paper made his eyes bleed. It was not a pouring out of blood, but a tear or two because his eyes were so red. Most books and magazines have an acid in the paper that he reacted to. I devised a plan to use a Pyrex roasting pan to cover the book and wooden tongs for him to turn the pages. I eventually discovered acid free paper so he could write. He could write with a pencil.

4. An incapability of eating/digesting anything inorganic or containing antibiotics or pesticides. He would not be able to keep anything down and he was losing weight rapidly.

We went to Whole Foods for meat and vegetables. His favorite daily eating was lamb steak, a baked potato and green beans. Sometimes Whole Foods' produce was marked "organic," but he would react negatively nevertheless. I turned to organic gardening to insure the pureness of the vegetables.

5. An allergic reaction to most cloth. He was unable to tolerate most clothes and would get rashes and an unbearable itching. I found organic alternatives online, including clothing and bedding and towels from Garnett Hill, and an organic duvet from a sheep ranch in British Columbia.

Bret's illness reminded me of the story of the Dutch Boy who put his finger in the hole in the dam to stop the water from pouring through. When he did that, however, a new hole would spring up, again and again, until he ran out of fingers. The futility of it all! And that was what Bret was experiencing—every time one "hole" (symptom) was contained, new "holes" would emerge.

MCS

Today, science and medicine have a name for what Bret experienced when he came into contact with chemicals: "Multiple Chemical Sensitivities."

· · ·

I like to think of it as an allergic reaction to chemicals, but I know this is a simplified explanation of a much more complicated reality.

What happens to the person with MCS is that he or she has a violent reaction to exposure to an external man-made chemical, causing the person's body to react negatively.

EMS

In 2010, when we researched what was happening to Bret with electricity and WIFI, we could only find one person— in Scotland, no less—who had similar symptoms. Today it is called "Electro Magnetic Sensitivity" (EMS, for short), also known as "Electromagnetic Hypersensitivity" (EHS), "EMF Aware," "EMF Injured," "Microwave or Radiation Sickness." They have conferences on this!

What happened to him when he was exposed to things such as High Tension Towers, WiFi and electricity in the home was that he experienced abdominal pain, brain fog, and chronic pain.

Losing the war

We had won a few battles but were losing the war. Bret is 6'3" and had been reduced to 87 pounds, had very dark circles under his eyes, and didn't have the strength to do more than lie in bed most of the day. In reality, he was dying!

Bret had adverse physical reactions to many household items that were toxic to him, and it got so bad we had to close off one room in the house for him. The room we selected had been used as our office and library and had a sliding glass door to give outside access. So everything had to be removed from the office to create Bret's new room. I took a lawn and leaf bag and systematically dragged the books down the hallway—as many as I could carry. Friends helped us move the big furniture from one room to the next. The door to the room was sealed off on both sides with rags and towels to prevent any negative chemical reactions. We had sealed Bret off as if he was "Bubble Boy."

Every morning I would use unbleached paper towels, and take a Sudoku book and pencil to transfer the puzzles onto the towels. I wanted to keep his mind active and transferred as many of these for him as possible. He could only drink, without reaction, Saratoga Water in the blue bottle with metal—not plastic—around the cap. The only food he could keep down was lamb steak from Whole Foods and some organic vegetables. All of his needs had to be brought around through the sliding glass door.

Since Bret was unable to go into the house, he was unable to use the bathroom. Ernie set up a camp potty for him and it was Ernie who maintained the space everyday, including cleaning it out and sanitizing it. I would bring him a bowl with water, Dr. Bronner's, and an organic washcloth so he could clean himself. He used organic toothpaste to brush his teeth.

Unfortunately, the Saratoga Water Company stopped manufacturing their water bottles with a metal ring, which were the only ones that Bret could drink from without an adverse reaction. Ernie and I went to every supermarket on Long Island to find the original bottles. I even called the company in Saratoga, New York to confirm that they changed the ring to plastic. Also, the Saratoga Water Company did not have any of the originals available at their warehouse.

One day his EMF reaction was so severe and his pain so great that Bret couldn't find peace in the house. His physical environment—despite our very best efforts to accommodate him—was killing him. He had to find another place to live!

. . .

My girlfriend Dorothy volunteered to have him stay at her house so off we went, hoping that a change of location would ease Bret's suffering. She had one of her sons vacate his room for Bret.

When he got there it was quickly discovered that he would not be able to stay. Her home was close to a high tension tower and some of the perfumes and colognes that were present in her house were making him sicker. This would not work either.

I ended up driving to my parents' home, in nearby Nassau County, trying to avoid the high tension towers as we went, and Bret found a spot at the foot of their bed where he could feel relief. He lay on the floor in a fetal position and was finally able to drift off to sleep.

It was a heart-wrenching scene that left me and my parents speechless. Speechless! But we still had to face the unanswered question: where would we go from here?

I would do whatever it took to get Bret healthy again. I was ready, determined—and I knew I had to be strong!

5

Meeting Dr. Sprouse

*A*fter much online searching, we found a doctor, Dr. Adrienne Sprouse, on Park Avenue in Manhattan and scheduled an appointment with her. Dr. Sprouse is a specialist in the field of environmental medicine, and is considered an expert in this field. She has been dealing with issues in environmental medicine since 1992, treating thousands of patients—adults and children alike—who have experienced illness as a result of environmental factors.

Driving Bret to his appointment in New York City was no easy task. He had extremely bad reactions to high tension towers, but we knew where every one of them existed on Long Island. By this time no maps necessary! But approaching Manhattan—further from our home than we were accustomed to traveling—meant entering an area with which we were less familiar. Bret said his reaction to these towers was as if someone were stabbing him repeatedly in his stomach with a sharp knife. He would scream in agony and writhe in pain when near one.

We learned how to navigate our destinations by trial and error. In other words, when Bret started writhing and shrieking in pain, saying "I can't take this," we would drive away from that location as quickly as possible. The worst spot on Long Island was Exit 53 on the LIE—the Long Island Expressway. We learned that because of the one time we brought him to my parents' house and he had a horrible reaction to that area. So to reach Dr. Sprouse's office in New York City, we would have to find yet another acceptable route back and forth on the highways.

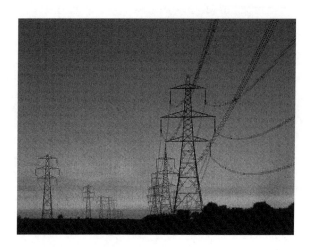

High tension towers

Mission accomplished! We would avoid Exit 53 by driving south on Nicolls Road, to Sunrise Highway west, then Sunrise Highway to Southern State Parkway west, then Southern State to the Seaford Oyster Bay Expressway north, and finally the Long Island Expressway west to the Midtown Tunnel into Manhattan.

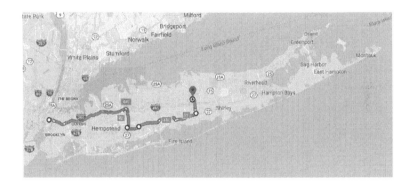

Our route to Manhattan, avoiding the high tension towers.

The day we went to New York City to meet with Dr. Sprouse, it was raining. I couldn't use the defrosters for the windows. Our solution was to bring a large roll of paper towels and continually wipe off the front windows. It was a huge challenge, but we made it!

Dr. Sprouse had an office on Park Avenue in Manhattan. Like her and her treatments, the office was very different from a conventional doctor's office. It looked like the office also served as her apartment; her dining area was used for group treatments and we waited to see her in a room that doubled as a living room. I couldn't help but think, "What rabbit hole did we fall into?" I found out later that all of us were thinking the same thing, but none of us spoke of it that day. Our only hope was that she could provide help.

Bret went in to see her first. Ernie and I waited. Then it was our turn.

I will never forget the picture that she drew to explain Bret's illness. She drew a picture of a funnel. She explained to us that Bret's liver had been compromised and likened what was happening in that organ to that funnel.

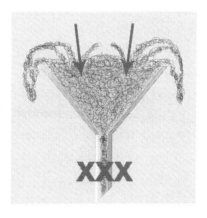

The arrows represent the toxins which should
be filtered through the liver. Due to the clog, the
toxins couldn't be filtered out, and instead
"spilled out" into Bret's body, causing all of
these adverse side effects.

Ordinarily the liver will flush out all toxins and chemicals in the body. As in the picture of that funnel, the toxins, chemicals, etc. go into the liver and are processed. What was happening to Bret was that his liver was clogged up and all of the toxins and chemicals were pouring into his body and not getting flushed out.

From her conversations with us, she diagnosed that Bret's illness was brought about by multiple exposures:

One was a negative reaction to Levaquin, an antibiotic he was prescribed for a urinary tract infection. (There was a class action suit on this drug, but Bret did not qualify because his tendons didn't explode.)

The other was probable exposure to black mold (scientific name: Stachybotrys chartarum), a microfungus that can be deadly to humans. Remember, Bret had lived off campus in Fairfax, Virginia while attending George Mason University. The apartment complex inhabited by the students—Camp Pyro—was filthy. Bret also told us that he had been sleeping on a mattress that he found in front of someone's home, waiting to be picked up by the sanitation department. Yuck! This explains a lot.

Dr. Sprouse also told us that she would be able to provide multiple treatments for Bret that would eventually open up the funnel and all would be fine. She couldn't promise how long it would take, but he would be better.

A game plan was established that included Bret coming to her office twice a week as well as the delivery of oxygen tanks that would be ordered for him for use in our house.

Dr. Sprouse never put a label on Bret's condition. (We found out the exact diagnosis later.) But more important than anything else—she said she could help! She said he would be better! She said he would be better!!

We were so thrilled! We would do anything to make that happen!

6

Getting Him Off the Grid

"*M*om, Dad, help me ease the pain I'm experiencing from the electricity in the house," Bret pleaded! We *had* to find a way to reduce the agony he was experiencing due to the extent of his EMS illness.

So we tried to develop a "game plan" that would help to ease Bret's suffering. The first step was to unplug the refrigerator in the kitchen. Who knew that an appliance could cause so much pain? The high electrical output and continual voltage from it was one of top culprits for my son's continual torture. So we unplugged it! But not for a few hours—all day, all night.

Ernie and I used coolers for the basics: milk, eggs, butter, etc. He was the cooler monitor. Translation, he made sure that there was always enough ice in the coolers so nothing would go bad. It was as if, like many years ago, we were camping.

We had no ice cube trays with ice, no ice cream, frozen foods, nor anything else in the house that must be kept frozen.

When we knew there were no urgent health issues occurring with Bret, Ernie and I would take an hour to eat out. We ate out a lot. There was a local diner so we could be close by, and my favorite was a nearby Mexican restaurant. There we could get paella and a pitcher of Sangria. Ice for our drinks was available in both locations.

Unplugging the refrigerator was a step in the right direction. It eased his discomfort a little bit, but he was still in continual pain. "Mom and Dad, please help me, please help me," said Bret.

We decided as our next step to shut down the electricity at night in the entire house. It was an electrical experiment to see how he would react. We hoped that the self-imposed blackout would help his pain. And it did!

Every evening we would set up for bed and then Ernie

would turn off every circuit in the house. We were off the grid!

Bret got relief and was able to sleep at night. A bit of a sacrifice, but a step in the right direction! If he could heal and recover from this shocking illness, it was worth it!

7

May, the Mold Lady

*O*ne of the tasks that we were asked to complete by Dr. Sprouse was to have our house inspected for black mold, or any other potentially harmful molds. In addition, we needed to have our home checked for the voltage levels coming into the house to determine if they may be too high. We were referred to May Dooley, a specialist in detecting and identifying molds and checking voltage in residences.

Since meeting with Dr. Sprouse, a whole new world had opened up to us. I never would have otherwise considered the effects of the electricity in our house, or that high voltages could harm us.

May lived in a remote, isolated area in Pennsylvania where she could distance herself from high voltages and harmful chemicals. She had similarly been exposed herself, and had dealt with symptoms like my son experienced. Once recovered, she stayed clear of any possible re-exposure by living away from all possible harmful external toxins that might cause her a relapse.

May came to our house one Saturday morning with equipment in tow. Devoted to helping others like her, she came out of her own place of safety to assist others—in this case, us. She set up her "laboratory" on our dining room table, placing her microscope at the head of the table (Ernie's seat).

She labeled different areas throughout the house and each station had a number. She swabbed each spot with a long cotton swab and then rolled the swabbing into a Petri dish. Each Petri dish was labeled with the same number as the location. Upstairs and downstairs she focused on locations where there might be mold.

I was her lab assistant! I followed her in the house and pointed out potential problem spots. It took all day to get samples, grow the dishes, review the growth under the microscope, then record the data. I helped with each part of the inspection.

While we were waiting for growth in the Petri dishes, May

brought out a voltage meter to measure the electricity in each room. She inspected our home again, room by room, for electrical surges—areas where the voltage may be too high.

Once she gave each dish adequate time to grow, she would study each dish under the microscope, identifying mold species, if any, growing in the dish. She showed me every dish and one by one discussed the results.

I was pleased to find out that our house was okay. No deadly molds, no high voltages. She did make a few recommendations, including buying a specific HEPA vacuum, and to have the electric company come and test our external wires for high voltage. Also, she asked us to remove all organic matter from the basement, i.e. clothes, paper, wood, etc. to prevent the possibility of future mold growth. We could keep all items made of glass, metal or plastic.

While our home was labeled safe for mold and electricity, however, Bret's initial exposure to mold at college and the negative reaction to Levaquin still left him sick. He still had to be isolated in the middle room. By having the house tested, at least we knew he still wasn't being exposed.

We complied with all of her recommendations! They made sense. We had to take whatever steps were necessary to get

Bret better! I felt a sense of relief and a firm conviction that we were moving in the right direction. Adrienne Sprouse, the environmental doctor, and May Dooley, the mold specialist, were moving Bret in a positive direction with a series of treatments that were unknown to us prior to meeting them.

8

Masks and Tanks

*B*ret went to New York City two days a week for appointments at Dr. Sprouse's office.

He would dress in black pants and a black hoodie with the hood on his head. He wore a filtered mask, the Sperian Saf-T-Fit Plus. The technical name for the mask was a "particulate respirator." We would order them from Grainger's and they worked well for him.

So Bret reminded me of the Unibomber!

Ernie drove him to the train station each Tuesday and Thursday for his appointments.

• • •

He would stay there for a number of hours, with a treatment plan that included chelation, vitamins, and sauna. Chelation, by the way, is a chemical process that is used to rid the body of excess or toxic metals. Medicines are introduced to the blood stream intravenously which attract the metals in the body, helping them to be flushed out.

Then Ernie would pick him up.

As per Dr. Sprouse's instructions, Bret required a supply of oxygen at the house. Bret wore the oxygen mask regularly, and once a month three large replacement oxygen tanks were delivered.

Also, Bret discovered at Dr. Sprouse's office that she had a water cooler he could drink from. The water was from Mountain Valley Spring Water; the distributor for our area was through Health Waters, Inc., in Carlstadt, New Jersey. I was able to order a ceramic dispenser from them that sat on a wooden base.

They also had big glass bottles in 2.5 and 5 gallon sizes. We set up a regular delivery schedule for the water, and they would drop off new bottles and pick up the used bottles for recycling.

. . .

We all used the water for drinking, cooking, coffee.

A new routine was in place!

9

Heating the Space

$\mathcal{F}$all was approaching as were the new challenges that cooler weather brings.

We hired an HVAC (heating, ventilation and air conditioning) specialist to seal off the air duct in Bret's room. He was unable to tolerate the heat blasting through the ducts.

It is amazing how often we take the simple things in life for granted. Now it seemed that Bret was becoming more alienated, more sealed off—and I was helpless to prevent it. All I could do was to figure out the next step to keep him alive, and not allow the despair to overtake me.

So how do you keep him warm?

• • •

I devised a plan where Ernie and Bret would leave after dinner to play a game of Scrabble at Whole Foods. Whole Foods has sections of tables and chairs for diners, and Bret and Ernie would secure a table to play one game. Bret was able to go to Whole Foods because they did not stock any harmful chemicals, detergents, cleaners, etc. That translated to no "off-gassing" in the store. Off-gassing occurs when new manufactured items release volatile organic compounds or chemicals.

As soon as they left, I would carry a few electric heaters around to the backyard and plug them in his room to heat up the area. Then I'd leave and go back around to the front of the house. Ernie would call when they were on their way home, and I reversed the process.

That meant racing around from our side door to the sliding glass door in the back of the house, unplugging the space heaters, closing the door quickly so the heat wouldn't escape his room, and carrying the heaters around the back to the side door. All while holding a flashlight!

It was particularly spectacular when there was a full moon that illuminated the entire backyard. I certainly didn't need a flashlight then! The light from the moon spotlit the entire backyard and filled my being with wonder and awe. It made everything seem small and gave me hope that Bret would be healed. It was a magical moment!

. . .

The moon is a strong magnetic force on the earth. The lunar phases control the waves and the tides, and perhaps, our behavior. The moon became my beacon of hope, my magnetic compass of strength.

It was also during a full moon that I had my "Scarlet O'Hara Moment": With a clenched fist in the air I declared to the universe, "As God as my witness, I will make this yard a garden of beauty, a celebration of nature!"

And I did!

However, winter was coming. What would we do then?

10

The Clara Moment

"*Mom* I feel better, I finally feel better!" Bret said the weekend before Thanksgiving 2010. Just as Dr. Sprouse had said, the "funnel" opened! Bret was feeling better!

My husband and I cried at this proclamation. Joy, happy joy to hear those words! It felt as if that proverbial black cloud had suddenly moved away. But was Bret cured? The three of us had the fear that his feeling better was only temporary.

We kept doing the same routine because we did not want to cause a relapse. At that time, Bret was still going to Dr. Sprouse two days a week, Ernie and Bret still went to Whole Foods while I heated up the room. We continued to turn off the power when we went to bed. Life continued.

Bret stayed in his sealed room, still cut off from the rest of the house.

But he was feeling better.

I was having Thanksgiving at our house and my parents were joining us. I suggested to Bret that he have his "grand opening" during Thanksgiving. He said "That sounds like a good idea."

So Thanksgiving arrived! It would be the five of us: me, Ernie, Mom, and Dad, and a sealed off Bret. We had turkey, mashed potatoes, stuffing, cranberry sauce, gravy, fresh broccoli and cauliflower and, of course, a can of Delmonte green beans for my Dad (he was never interested in fresh vegetables so it became a running family joke). It was topped off with one of my homemade apple pies, a family favorite.

I was anxious during the entire meal, wondering if he was ready to take that giant step, to open the door. Was he ready physically and emotionally?

We retired to the living room to digest that huge meal. Much of the conversation focused on Bret—how he was, how he was feeling. I was very nervous that he wouldn't open the door today, that his fears would get the best of him. After all, it was a huge step. It also was getting late and Thanksgiving was almost over. Suddenly, we all heard the middle room door open and Bret came out into the living room! He broke the seal and moved all of the protective insulation blocking the door. It was a miracle!

The moment we all dreamed of had come!

A cheer arose from the four of us! There wasn't a dry eye in the house! Sobs! It was emotionally overwhelming!

It reminded me of the film *Heidi*, starring Shirley Temple. There is a scene where they are celebrating Christmas. (Ok, ours was Thanksgiving.) Heidi and her friend Clara, who is in a wheelchair, had been working every day to get her to walk. At Christmas dinner, Heidi and Clara showed Clara's father that Clara was able to walk, when she got up and walked to her father. There wasn't a dry eye in the house.

Sound familiar? We had our Clara moment.

Part Two

The Spiritual Journey

Magic

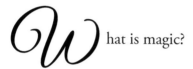hat is magic?

The English Oxford Living Dictionary defines the word as follows:

Noun

1. The power of apparently influencing events by using mysterious or supernatural forces.

1.1 Mysterious tricks, such as making things disappear and reappear, performed as entertainment.

1.2 A quality of being beautiful and delightful in a way that seems remote from daily life. "The magic of theatre"

1.3 Exceptional skill or talent.

Adjective

1. Having or apparently having supernatural powers.

1.1 Very effective in producing the desired results

2. Wonderful, exciting.

Verb

1. Move, change or create by or as if by magic.

To the surprise and shock of all of us, Bret had emerged from the room with seemingly magical abilities. He seemed to be able to communicate with spirits and had psychic abilities.

One vivid example of this was when he suddenly said to me, "Grandma says thank you."

I said, "What do you mean? Is it Grandma Springer or Grandma Weissman?"

He said "You know."

"What do you mean—I know."

He said "You know."

He was getting me annoyed, but at the same time, he was triggering me to think.

"Bret, can't you give me a clue?" I said.

"You know," he said.

And suddenly it came to me—I knew!

A few weeks before, I was looking for photos for my parents' upcoming anniversary party to use for a video montage.

In their wedding album was a photo I never saw before. It was my Mom on her wedding day, in her wedding gown, flanked by my two Grandmothers. MY FEMALE ROOTS!

I was so excited by this photo that I made two prints of it and framed them, one for me, one for my Mom. I even posted the picture on Facebook.

It was the only photo of my Grandma Weissman that was framed and displayed in any of the households, thus bringing her image back to the family.

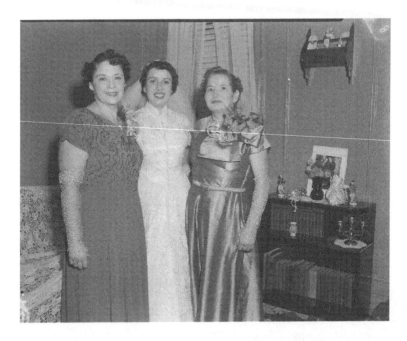

Grandma Springer, Mom and Grandma Weissman

I got it! I got a message from Grandma Weissman!

Bret became an avid reader of motivational and spiritual books.

The first book he recommended was *Being in Balance, 9 Principles For Creating Habits to Match Your Desires,* by Dr. Wayne W. Dyer.

Bret said, "Here!" and handed me the book.

· · ·

What a revelation! What a joy! And the quotes he cited inspired me.

Since then, I have been a huge fan of Wayne Dyer, re-reading the book numerous times, watching his PBS specials, reading his other books and listening to his tapes. Rest In Peace, Wayne.

The other book he gave me to read was *An Open Heart, Practicing Compassion in Everyday Life*, by the Dalai Lama. In Chapter 7 of the book he writes: "What is Compassion? Compassion is the wish that others be free of suffering. It is by means of Compassion that we aspire to attain an enlightenment."

Bret had become my guru!

12

Out the Door, but not Out of the Woods

*B*ret was physically on track again. He was no longer in the sealed room, no longer electromagnetic sensitive, and no longer having severe reactions to chemicals.

However, mentally and emotionally he was a wreck! He had developed some completely understandable fears— and justifiably so! He was afraid of how he might react to different chemicals, or anything else, for that matter.

Could there be even one thing out there that might push him over the edge and back into the isolation room, back to 87 pounds, back to near death—or maybe this time to death itself?

. . .

Bret began to explore his options explored options and found Colleen Flanagan, while searching online, who specializes in a form of counseling intervention   called "EFT". She resides in Arizona, and Bret was able to have individual phone sessions with her a few times a week.

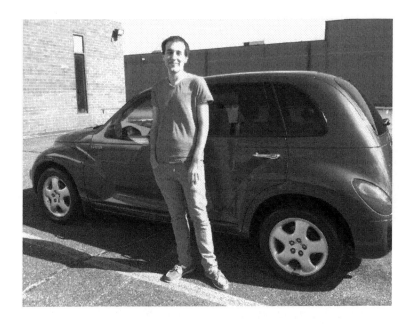

Bret and his PT Cruiser

Colleen introduced Bret to Emotional Freedom Technique (EFT), also known as "tapping", which harnesses the energy system in a person's body. It is a self-help technique that was developed first by Dr. Roger Callahan and later modified by energy pioneer Gary Craig, where the person "taps" near the end points of his/her "energy meridians" to stimulate the body's own healing powers. Tapping is also referred to as "Psychological Accupuncture." Normally, these meridian pathways are open, but when we have fears, stress, pain, etc., we create blockages in our pathways. The tapping technique frees the body's energy flow. One of the major fringe benefits of EFT is that the technique is free of medications, equipment or supplements.

And EFT—happily—worked for Bret! He was able to conquer his fears and get back to a balanced, fearless life.

After his physical recovery, Bret stayed at our house for one more month because our home brought up too many painful memories for him. Lurking in the background was always the fear that something in the house would trigger a reaction that would catapult him back into his isolation room.

So, as 2011 began, Bret moved in with my parents for 6 months. It was tax season, and Dad always needed help with the tax returns. My son was quite eager to make some money for the first time since his illness. It was a good start for him as Dad's apprentice.

Bret made his bed on their living room couch, and slept accompanied by my parents' dog, Lola.

This was a step in the right direction, but only one step on a much longer journey. Bret wanted more!

13

Reconnecting to the Earth

One of the processes that helped Bret during his severe bout of EMS was grounding, also known as "earthing." It refers to direct contact with the Earth's surface by such means as walking barefoot outside, strolling on the beach, laying prone on the ground, or gardening. The direct contact passes the electrical current into the ground, in the same way as a lightning rod grounds or an electrical appliance employs an electrical outlet.

Bret would also get a similar grounding effect by placing his hands around a tree trunk. So tree hugging became a medicinal practice for him. There was one particular large White Maple in our backyard that was most effective. Sad to say, that tree lost its life during Super Storm Sandy.

As I promised, when I was going around the backyard

every evening to heat his room, I intended to turn our yard into an oasis of beauty. To accomplish this, lots of work and planning had to be done. Each bed around my house was measured and the plants used were planned. I purchase the Moleskine Gardening Journal each year to plan and record the year's planting journey, and I take photos of the season's plants. (You may have seen some of my photos on Facebook with my "Greeting from the Garden" postings.) This helps me determine next year's crop.

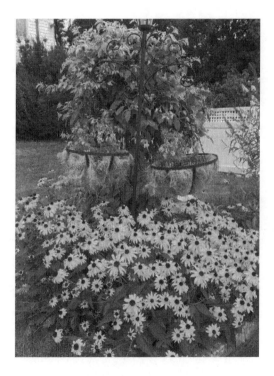

Black-eyed Susans

Although he did not live with us in the spring, Bret would come often to visit. He was truly grounded to the earth, and we would make it a point, especially in the spring, to be out in the backyard.

The organic gardening I had started to do on a small scale when he was ill "blossomed" into a larger garden the spring of 2011. We all enjoyed the vegetables, herbs and fruits from the garden, especially tomatoes, strawberries, garlic, rosemary, oregano, basil, cucumbers, radishes and the greens.

In going organic there are three essentials to begin with:

• Organic Potting Soil or Organic Top Soil

• Organic Seeds or Seedlings

• Organic Mulch, Compost or Peat Moss

You can check online for the availability of organic soils, mulch, compost, or peat moss in hardware stores or organic farms.

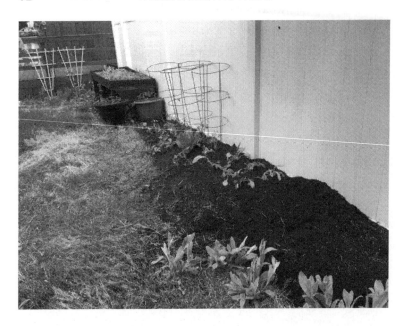

Seedlings in my vegetable garden.

I found my organic seeds online at Botanical Interests, Territorial Seed and Renee's Garden. These seed companies have organic and regular seeds, so make sure your purchase has the organic label. For organic seedlings, my favorite company is Mountain Valley Growers.

There are multiple choices and options for seeds, plants, soils, and tools, so I found my best resources by trial and error.

A bird feeder was a valuable and fun addition to the back-yard. It was exciting to observe the different bird species. I placed the feeders on the other side of the yard so it also kept the birds away from the garden. A proverbial win-win.

One day, Bret and I were sitting in the backyard, talking and watching the birds. All of a sudden we heard a loud flapping of wings. A red-tailed hawk, a carnivore, was making an attempt to have lunch at the bird feeder. It was a failed attempt as I had placed the feeders in the corner of the fence. The hawk's wingspan was too wide to get by the feeders. Saved!

And Bret was saved, too. He was now ready to begin his journey to explore the spiritual possibilities that would ultimately complete him.

14

Church of the Metaphysical Science

*B*ret and I were sitting at the dining room table when Bret said, in a voice deeper and different than his speaking voice, "I would like to introduce myself, my name is Zedekiel and I am your Guardian Angel!"

I did a double-take and said to Bret, "What did you say?" He said, "I didn't say anything."

This was amazing, and so nice to meet my Guardian Angel, and I immediately went to research who he was, as I had never heard of the name Zedekiel before. Another magical event.

According to the *Zohar*, which is the holy book of the mystical branch of Judaism known as Kabbalah, Zedekiel is an Archangel, known for being the Archangel of freedom, benevolence and forgiveness. Tradition considers him to be the Angel of Mercy, and he is often thought to be the angel who stopped the Patriarch Abraham from sacrificing his son Isaac. The name Zedekiel is a Hebrew name usually translated as the "righteousness of God."

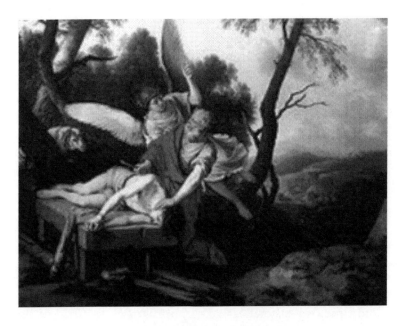

Zedekiel, the Archangel

I found myself doing a lot of research lately as many new and wonderful events were happening before me. I was now a researcher of things metaphysical and spiritual!

Bret became a member of the Church of the Metaphysical Science at this time. Located in Patchogue, the Church of the Metaphysical Science focuses on spiritualism and mediumship. It is a chartered church of the National Spiritualistic Association of Churches.

Bret was involved with them for about six months.

Their service was on Sundays at 11 AM, and I accompanied him on several occasions. The first time I went, a gentleman came up to me and said, "Your son is the real deal!" I didn't know the man, and I never saw him again. He was referring to Bret's psychic ability.

Every time I attended services, I received a message. When one of the ministers had a message for you, he or she would ask, "Would you like to receive a message?" I always said, "Yes!"

One time, my sister-in-law, Mary, came with Bret and me to the Sunday service. She was asked if she would like to receive a message, and, of course, she said "Yes."

"There is a woman you once knew, famous for making apple pies, who wants to tell you that you have turned out to be a very nice woman," said the minister.

· · ·

Mary and I looked at each other in surprise and disbelief! There was an older woman, Mrs. Meeney, who lived next door to her parents when they retired to Jay, New York. She would always bake her famous apple pies when any of us came upstate for a visit.

It could only be her! We were both amazed and impressed. A "hair-raising" moment!

I was also told that I had a "brain full of knowledge" that I had to teach to others. How profound a statement!

15

Access Consciousness

"*I* have a wonderful story to tell you," said Mary G. as I entered her basement apartment.

I had come to get my Access Consciousness certification, and she was my instructor. To backpedal slightly, Bret had become acquainted with a series of techniques and processes called Access Consciousness, which had a major impact on him. It's purpose is to empower individuals to create the lives they desire. It sets out to offer step-by-step techniques and tools to enable practitioners to become more conscious in everyday life, and to eliminate barriers preventing people from truly living fulfilling lives.

In Access Consciousness, a process called "running the bars" involves a person touching various parts of another's head, which helps to release the energies trapped there.

Different touch points on the head are connected to different receptors, such as creativity, energy and relationships. The "head" is the person who is being touched—generally while lying face up—while the other person is standing above, gently pressing and releasing the energies from their head.

Bret had asked me to get certified. This required me to attend an eight-hour class that included a video, demonstrations and practice. Mary asked her sister to join us to be the 'head' for the class.

"It was your son Bret who came to my apartment to train me! He was living in Brooklyn and had to take the Long Island Railroad and a cab to get here. It was a long trip. Needless to say, he immediately went to use the bathroom in my house."

When he came out he announced, "Mary, there is a female spirit in your bathroom. She is standing in the corner." I told Bret that my mother had recently died and it must have been her. We went into the bathroom together and told her it was okay to go. And she did! "Your son holds a special place in my heart!" Mary exclaimed.

When Bret first discovered Access Consciousness, he found

his home, but he had to practice on someone to improve his skills, so he picked me to be his "head!"

The first time he "ran the bars," the terminology of the energy clearing, it took about 1 1/2 hours.

When it was completed, Bret and I went out on the upper deck of our house to get a breath of fresh air and to talk about the experience. When we looked to our right we saw a double rainbow in the sky! Wow! It was a validation from the universe.

Bret gave Ernie and me a book to read, *Being You, Changing the World* by Dr. Dain Heer, one of the co-founders of Access Consciousness. I recommend it to anyone who wishes to explore this further.

Access Consciousness has opened doors for Bret—one door that includes traveling all over the world. He also met his soulmate, Georgia, at an Access Consciousness conference in Washington State. He truly found the perfect path for his life.

16

Brooklyn

---

*B*ret decided to "spread his wings" and get his own place to live in Brooklyn, the "in" place to be. He shared two apartments that didn't work out due to the roommates or the location. Around the same time, Georgia moved from Oregon to Brooklyn. When his shared apartments didn't work out, Georgia offered Bret the use of her art studio for his apartment. Eventually, he moved into her apartment.

I was able to visit with them more frequently! I would pick them up at their storefront apartment in Carroll Gardens and drive across the bridge to Soho.

Bret, Georgia and I would have a grand day in Soho! Walking, exploring, shopping, eating. Our favorite place to have dinner was Pepolino's, a well-reviewed Italian restaurant on West Broadway in TriBeCa. It was magical to be together!

Ernie would eventually join us.

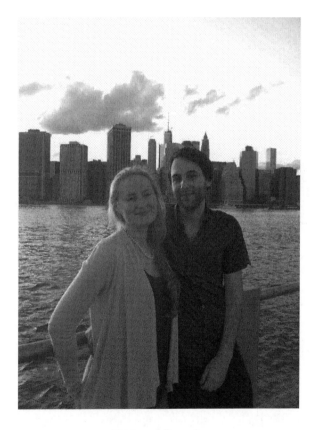

Bret and Georgia

In July, on our wedding anniversary, we scheduled a "Soho day!" And it was perfect, ending the day with an anniversary dinner at Pepolino's.

· · ·

We dropped Bret and Georgia off at their apartment and, as we were saying our goodbyes, Bret said, "Oh by the way...Georgia and I have decided to move to Houston. We are moving in two weeks." Truthfully, we didn't see that coming! Why Houston? It is so far away? The co-founders of Access Consciousness live in Houston, so I suppose I shouldn't have been surprised by Bret's move there. Why the rush to be gone in two weeks? Confusion, disappointment and shock were all grappling to take center stage in our hearts.

That was our last Soho Day.

17

Houston, the Eagle Has Landed

I got a call from Bret and the conversation began, "Hi, Mom. I am getting on the plane to Houston in 10 minutes…"

Before he could say anything else or before I could hear anything else, I lost it and broke down and cried. Sobbing! Crying as I have never cried! Releasing all of the crying I had held back during all of the previous chapters in our life. I moved the phone away from my ear, my arm outstretched as far as it could go. Even then I wanted to protect him and I wanted to be strong.

But it was uncontrollable. As I valiantly attempted to compose myself, I brought the phone back to my ear and croaked (sort of a croak). It was important to get back into the conversation as I was wasting the few minutes we had before he got on the plane.

He was surprised at my response. He could hear it, and said "Mom, why are you so upset? This is what we worked for. This is what you told me when all was at its darkest, that I had to fight, fight, fight, so I could be independent and free!"

And he was right! At times when he was at his darkest, when he was struggling, I often reminded him that he had to fight to be independent and free, to be healthy and cured, so he could have the lifestyle he wanted.

I told him, still choking back my tears, "Yes I know. Then why does it hurt so much?"

He thanked me for everything, and he and Georgia got on the plane, on their way to Houston, Texas, to a new life and independence!

Part Three

A Resource Guide

18

A Resource Guide

*T*his is a list of the resources that provided comfort and solutions for my son during his illness, products that supported our family before and after his illness and recovery to health.

It is my intention to help you on your journey.

May Dooley

www.createyourhealthyhome.com

Mold testing and Electromagnetic Field testing

May was recommended by Dr. Sprouse. She came to our home and tested for toxic molds and high voltage in our house.

Mountain Valley Spring Water

www.mountainvalleyny.com

Water delivery service providing water in glass bottles from 1 liter to 5 gallons.

Dr. Sprouse had the five gallon bottles, supported by a wooden holder, in her office. We ordered the 5-gallon bottles and the wooden support. The truck would come to Long Island once a week, pick up the empties for recycling, and drop off new bottles.

Multiple Chemical Sensitivity: Herbal and Nutritional Remedies

Facebook Group

https://www.facebook.com/groups/1467877260150671/

This site discusses current questions and health issues pertaining to MCS and EMS.

. . .

I discovered this group once Bret's illness had been healed. My cousin, JMe Isman manages this Facebook group. I had found out around a month after Bret's healing that she too was living with MCS and EMS.

Her site contains an invaluable list of environmental doctors located in the United States.

Our Little Place

www.ourlittleplace.com

Information about Environmental Illness, Multiple Chemical Sensitivity, Chronic Fatigue Syndrome, Lyme Disease, the health risks of perfume, fabric softeners, and air fresheners, and guidelines for nontoxic living.

This was the first website we found that spoke in depth about Bret's health issues. We used this site when Bret was first diagnosed to get information and answers.

Rawganique

www.rawganique.com

Products that are pesticide-free, GMO-free, and free of other chemicals and dyes.

Bret was able to find clothes he could wear and bedding he could sleep on. One of the items he ordered was organic Long Johns.

Rawganique also provided acid free paper and journals! So he was able to write again! Their products were liberating for him.

Eco-Socks for NWP

www.ecosocks@wildernessproject.org

Organization that focuses on environmental restoration. They are no longer fundraising.

• • •

Bret was able to purchase socks that he didn't react to and were comfortable. The socks were organic and dye-free.

Garnet Hill

www.garnethill.com

Specializing in women's and children's clothing and household goods. Organic cotton and eco-merino wool are among the materials used in their products.

I ordered an organic fleece blanket and throw from Garnet Hill.

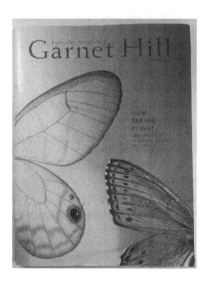

Emotional Freedom Technique

(EFT)

Colleen Flanagan

www.emorescue.com

EFT (tapping) resource located in Arizona.

We found Colleen online. Using EFT (Tapping), she was able to help Bret through his emotional fears.

Diane Gordon

www.yourthrivingrite.com

Based in Suffolk County, Long Island, New York, Diane teaches EFT (Tapping) and other energy modalities.

Eileen Lichtenstein

www.balanceandpower.com

Located in Nassau County, Long Island, New York, Eileen is your peak performance success coach for your life, career and family.

Masks and Filters

I Can Breathe

www.icanbreathe.com

A company that specializes in filtered breathing masks that are latex-free, reusable and washable.

We were able to get Bret a honeycomb mask and carbon filter refills for the mask.

Grainger

www.grainger.com

Industrial supplies and safety products for businesses.

This is where we ordered the Saf-T-Fit Plus Particulate Respirator, his first mask.

Oxygen Tanks

Apria Healthcare

www.apria.com

This is the company that delivered oxygen tanks to the house.

Since Bret was sealed in his room, the delivery man had to go around the backyard and up the stairs, through the sliding glass door to deliver the tanks.

Organic Seeds and Plants

Botanical Interests

www.botanicalinterests.com

Territorial Seed

www.territorialseed.com

Renee's Garden

www.reneesgarden.com

These three seed companies were where I purchased organic seeds for my home garden.

. . .

Mountain Valley Growers

www.mountianvalleygrowers.com

Organic perennial, vegetable and herb plants for sale.

An amazing company for purchasing seedlings, especially lavender. You get to learn both the common and Latin names of the plants for sale.

Gardening Supplies

Gardener's

www.gardeners.com

A good resource for gardening supplies and accessories.

A source for every gardening challenge, providing education and advice.

I purchased my VegTrug, my hose, etc. from this company.

Church of the Metaphysical Science

www.tmsli.org

It is the Mission of the Temple of Metaphysical Science, a chartered church of the National Spiritualist Association of Churches, to teach and proclaim the science, philosophy and religion of Spiritualism, which is the religion of continuous life, based on the demonstrated fact of communication, by means of mediumship, with those who live in the spirit world.

Bret worked with the members of the church. This experience helped him in his recovery.

Access Consciousness

www.accessconsciousness.com

Learning new and life-changing techniques, tools and processes that are designed to empower you. Practical, dynamic, and pragmatic, it provides step-by-step processes to facilitate you in being more conscious in every day life and eliminate all the barriers you have put up to receiving.

· · ·

Bret found his home and way of life discovering Access Consciousness. He works with Access, traveling all over the world.

Dr. Adrienne Sprouse

Found on WebMD and YouTube

Doctor specializing in Environmental Medicine.

Bret's Doctor who helped him get his health back. She gave us hope!

Books

Being In Balance, 9 Principles For Creating Habits To Match Your Desires, by Dr. Wayne W. Dyer.

An Open Heart, Practicing Compassion In Everyday Life, by the Dalai Lama.

Being You, Changing the World, by Dr. Dain Heer.

. . .

Birds, A Spiritual Field Guide, by Arin Murphy-Hiscock.

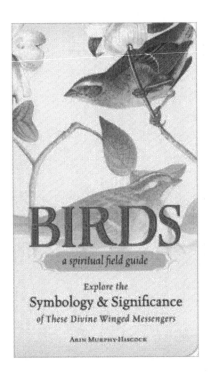

National Audubon Society Field Guide To The Mid-Atlantic States, the Chanticleer Press.

Epilogue

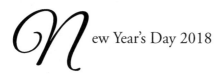ew Year's Day 2018

For years I had told others who asked about Bret's condition and recovery that, "You'll read about it in my book," but while I had several starts to my book, my writing had stalled.

When I got up on New Year's Day morning I opened the shades and looked out of the bedroom window. I saw something unusual on the branch of the spruce tree directly in front of that window. It almost looked like a plastic grocery store bag stuck in the tree.

. . .

I got my binoculars, and lo and behold, I was looking at a small reddish owl sleeping in the tree! I screamed so loud at the sight of this beautiful animal that I actually woke it up! (Being nocturnal, an owl will sleep during the day).

I woke Ernie to come and see the owl, got my camera, and got my Audubon Mid-Atlantic Field Guide to identify the owl. I was able to identify the bird as the Eastern Screech Owl (Megascops asio), the rufous color variety.

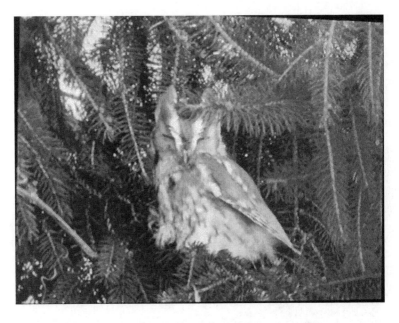

The Eastern Screech Owl, rufous color variety

Symbolically and spiritually, what does the owl mean? I got out my book, *Birds, a Spiritual Field Guide* by Arin Murphy-Hiscock. In Ancient Greece, the owl symbolized wisdom, as it was associated with Athena. I also Googled the symbolism of the Owl. The descriptions that resonated the most with me were that the owl symbolizes that "spirits are strong around you" and "it is the epitome of mystery, magic, vision, and guidance." So the owl is a messenger, a harbinger of magic and mysticism.

Murphy-Hiscock went on to say that "It is also one of the most ancient signs for spirit contact. The owl is the silent guide, teaching us to trust our instincts and silent impressions, especially in regards to spirit communication. Its appearance now is alerting you to much spirit activity around you."

I had to get a picture of that beautiful owl, so I brought out the iPad, but I was still unabe to get the picture that I wanted.

Then I brought out "Baby", my good camera—the Vivitar that I bought for our trip to Paris.

Poised at the window, camera at hand, I went to take the photo and nothing happens. THE BATTERY WAS DEAD! NO! Now I had to find the charger and charge the battery (the forces were against me to get a photo of this owl). I was concerned he would leave!

. . .

So after breakfast, I went back to see if he was still there and he was!! I had charged enough juice in the battery to get a few good shots. Hooray!

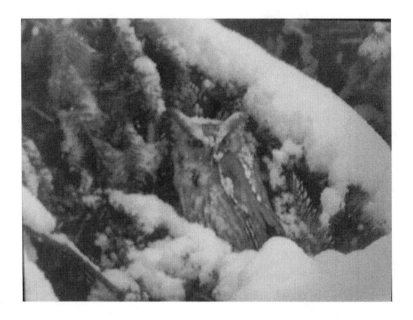

In order to get a good shot downloaded, you have to:

Connect to a computer

Download the photo

Email the photo to yourself

Save the photo to your iPad

Post to Facebook

. . .

I did not want to take the time to do this, so I took a photo with my iPad of the camera's viewing screen. It came out well! I was able to get a photo of him awake (remember I woke him with all of my hooting and hollering!)

I watched the owl all day! He did go back to sleep, looking like a rufous puffball in his resting pose. His chest was all puffed out. His chest reminded me of meringue, creamy color with peaks of darker brown.

The owl was there all day!

As dusk was approaching, I had the sense that my time with the owl would end soon. Around 4:45 pm he woke up from his sleep and moved his head as only an owl can (or the girl from *The Exorcist!*) I saw the bird move two steps to his left—and I knew our time together was up! And sure enough, he took off, quickly, without fanfare, and not as majestically as I thought it would look. Poof, he was gone!

That night, I fell asleep in front of the television at about 8 PM but awoke at about 10:20 PM. What impressed me when I awoke was that the kitchen was illuminated. What was that?

. . .

I looked out the side window to see an enormous full moon! Full moon!! I didn't know until then that there was a full moon that evening!

New Year's Day! Owl! Full moon! OMG!

Within minutes of seeing the moon and processing all of the blatant symbolism, the phone rang and it was Bret!

We had a great conversation without any distractions. I told him what happened today and, of course, he wasn't surprised.

Then we spoke about the recovery part of this book. I was able to interview him and clarify some timeline questions I had. It was liberating!

"Bret, do you want to contribute to the book?" I asked. He said, "Mom, this is your story, your perspective."

When I got off the phone I went back to the book and began to write. I began to outline the recovery section on MindMap.

. . .

My writer's block had ended. I was on my way again.

Thank you to the Owl, the Moon and my son Bret!

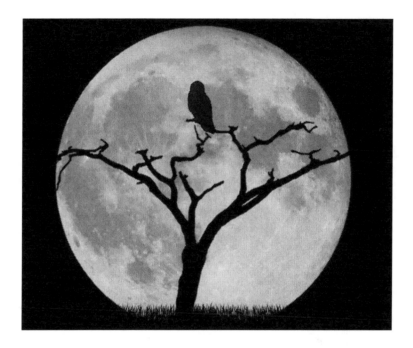

About the Author

Linda Springer, a native Long Islander, is a naturalist who was a curator and project developer at the Museum of Long Island Natural Sciences at SUNY Stony Brook. During her tenure, she co-authored three books, *A Field Guide to Long Island's Woodlands*, *A Field Guide to Long Island's Wetlands*, and *A Field Guide to Long Island's Seashore*.

Having worked in her parents' tax preparation business from the age of eight, Linda is an advocate for financial literacy. She is also skilled and experienced in personal finance.

Linda recently celebrated her 40th Wedding Anniversary with husband Ernie. An organic gardener, Linda loves shell collecting, bird watching, photography, cooking, and old movies. She excels in trivia.

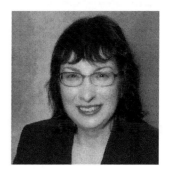

Made in the USA
Columbia, SC
08 November 2019